JN194646

宇城道塾の手引き

〈実践編①〉

身体に気を流す

宇城式呼吸法

宇城道塾事務局 編

宇城憲治 監修

はじめに

本来の身体のあるべき状態とは

道塾の手引き〈基本編〉では、宇城道塾で学ぶにあたっての基本心得や基本コンセプト、宇城憲治塾長のものの見方、考え方、生きざまなどを紹介いたしました。

〈実践編〉では、生まれながらに持つ身体の潜在力を発揮させるための基本的な実践プログラムを紹介していきます。その①として紹介するのが宇城式呼吸法です。

この呼吸法は、身体を自由に居つかずに使うための鍛錬法です。鍛錬法と言っても、一般のエクササイズのように、これをしたら身体に気が通るようになる、というようなハウツー的なものではなく、あくまでも身体本来のあり方に戻し、整えるために行なうものです。

そもそも私たちの身体は、常に気が流れ、身体の呼吸ができていることが本来の姿であり、むしろ、そのことに気づいてもらうためのプログラムであると考えてもらったほうがよいと思います。

「教える・学ぶ」から「気づく・気づかせる」の学び

道塾の学びはすべて、「自分の身体を通して、すなわち体感を通じて気づいていく」ことに徹しています。従来の学校教育や各種セミナーなどでは、まず教師が「教え」て、生徒が「学ぶ」というスタイルですが、このあり方だと、一方向の teaching の世界となり、生徒側は常に「頭で知識を受け取る」だけの受け身となってしまいます。道塾では自分の身体で能動的に理解することを大切にしています。

また本書シリーズで展開する「理論と実践」は、あくまでも「実証先にありき」の事実、実践に基づくものであります。宇城塾長によると、今の科学的な分析や文献は、この「実証先にありき」からすると、あまりに矛盾に満ちていると言います。道塾では、そうした分析や文献を実際に検証することで、その矛盾や理屈を浮き彫りにしつつ、同時にこれまで積み上げてきた実証事実を根拠としながら講義を展開していきます。

道塾において宇城塾長は常々、「人間は、自動車や飛行機やパソコンといった、設計図があって部品を組み合わせればできる物とは違い、どんな科学をもってしても、あるいは

世界のノーベル賞受賞者が集まったとしても、つくることができないものであり、かつ宇宙の創造物として神秘としか言いようがないものである」と言っています。

その神秘である人間の「生まれながらに持つ潜在力」や「可能性」を、今の常識ではあり得ない実践を通して体感し、それらを自分の中に取り戻すこと、これこそがこの道塾の大切な学びであるのです。それは知識で学んで身につくものではありません。

どんなに頭で「できない」「あり得ない」と思っても、自分の身体で「できて」しまえば、自分でそれを認めざるを得ません。それが次へのステップにつながる「気づき」であり、学びの原動力となります。その理屈抜きの「気づき」のきっかけが道塾の実践にあるのです。

本書「実践編 呼吸法」が様々な気づきの一助となることを願っています。

宇城道塾事務局

身体に気を流す　宇城式呼吸法　◎　目次

第一章　身体の呼吸とは

身体の呼吸とは

基本編で述べたように、道塾で言う「呼吸」とは、一般的な「口や鼻で吸って吐いて」の呼吸ではなく、身体で行なう呼吸のことを指します。

口や鼻での「吸って吐いて」の呼吸は生命体にとっては何よりも重要な呼吸であり、なかでも睡眠時の呼吸はもっとも自然体の無意識の呼吸で、それに代わる方法はありません。

一方で意識的に吸ったり吐いたりする色々な呼吸法がありますが、道塾で学ぶ呼吸法は、そうした呼吸法とは本質を異にします。道塾において塾生は宇城塾長が独自に修得した気というエネルギーによって様々な「今の常識ではあり得ない力や身体動作」を体験しますが、宇城式呼吸法はまさにそうした力を自ら生み出すベースとなる呼吸法です。さらにこの呼吸法は武術の極意にも通じる呼吸法であります。

武術のような、相手との攻防の状況に際しては、身体が居付いたり、固まったり、浮いたりすれば、それが即、命の危機に直結します。

身体が居付く、固まる、浮くということは身体の呼吸が止まっている状態であり、その身体は部分体となり、意識している部位以外は隙となり、周りに対して大変無防備な状態

となります。武術ではそれは即命取りとなります。

こうした命取りともなりかねない身体の状態から自らを守る身体すなわち統一体をつくる呼吸、そして自分の中にエネルギーを生み出す呼吸、それが本書で紹介する宇城式呼吸法です。

日常で起こる身体の居付きによる弊害

身体が居付いたり身体の呼吸が止まったりすることは、自身では気づいていないかも知れませんが、日常でひんぱんに起こります。そして居付いたり呼吸が止まったりすることからくる身体の不自由さ、無防備さは日常生活の中でも様々な弊害をもたらします。

何かに驚いたり、あせったり、あわてたりすると、気持ちが不安定となり身体はとたんに居付いた状態となり、身体の呼吸も滞ってしまいます。このような状態の時は、武術では隙となり危険です。またこの状態は、事故などにあった場合、大怪我につながったり、スポーツでは怪我につながり、仕事ではミスや不備、さらには人間関係のトラブルなど、あらゆることにもつながっていきます。

そのような状態から身を守り、さらには身体本来の力を発揮するためには、身体が居付かず自然体で、かつ意識からも自由であることが必須であり、それには、身体に「気が流れている」ことが大切です。

「身体に気が流れている」とは、**身体が本来の状態にあるということです。**すなわち自然体かつ強くしなやかな状態であり、植物が大地から養分をもらって成長するように、人間も大地とつながって、そこから得たエネルギーを伝える状態になるというものです。

呼吸による身体の変化

この「身体に気が流れている状態」は、「身体に気が流れていない状態」を体験すると、その違いがよくわかります。ですからまず、身体の呼吸が通った状態と、そうでない状態がどう異なるかを検証し、その体験を通して理解しておく必要があります。

「身体の呼吸が止まった状態」とは、単に口や鼻で息を吸ったり吐いたりする呼吸を止めている状態ではなく、例えば腕相撲などで相手を倒そうと力を入れた瞬間に、身体がぐっ

と固まるような状態を言います。

この状態になると呼吸が止まり、かつ身体の気も止まります。その事によって身体が固まり、居付きが生じ非常にもろくなります。その証拠に、その状態の時に腹や背中を叩かれたりすると、強い痛みを感じます。これは検証してみるとはっきりと体感することができます。

以下の検証は、『気の開発メソッド初級編』や『心と体 つよい子に育てる躾』などの本でも紹介している例ですが、「きちんと礼をする」ことで身体に気が通り、身体の呼吸ができている状態となります。そうすると以下のような様々な変化を体感することができます。

呼吸による身体の 変化Ⓐ 重くなる

① 二人一組になり、一人が相手を後ろから持ち上げます。簡単に持ち上がってしまいます。自分で「重くなれ」と頭で念じても結果は同じです。

② 今度は、①で持ち上げられた人が、相手に向かってきちんと礼をします。

③そして①と同じようにまた後ろからその人を持ち上げます。今度は持ち上げられないほど重くなっています。

① 持ち上がる

② きちんと礼をする

③ 持ち上がらない

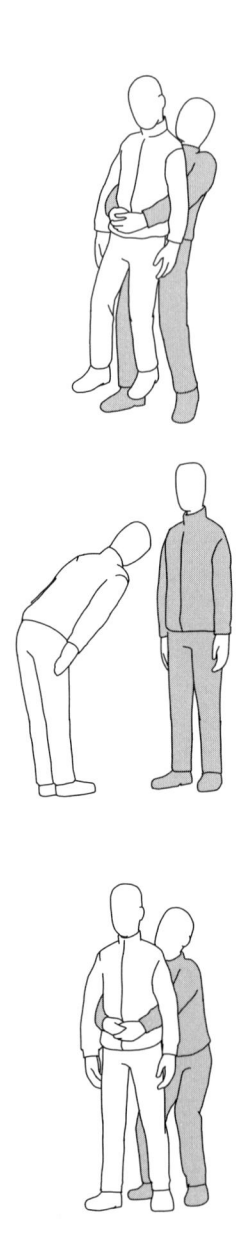

呼吸による身体の 変化B 強くなる

変化Aと同じく礼をする検証で、③の時に、後ろから持ち上げてもらうかわりに、相手に腕をつかんでもらいます。すると相手を簡単に投げることができます。

同じく③の時に、相手に腕を思いっきり叩いてもらいます。痛みはほとんど感じません。

むしろ叩いた人が手に痛みを感じるほど、身体は強くなっています。

② きちんと礼をする

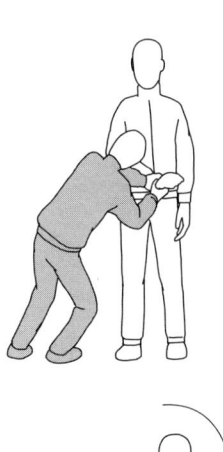

③-1 腕を掴まれる

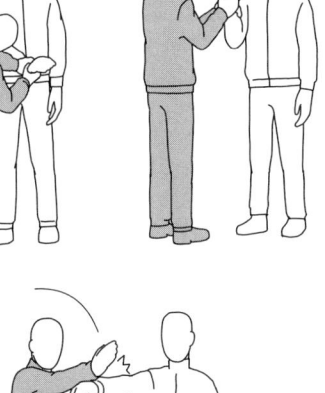

③-2 腕を思いきり叩いてもらう

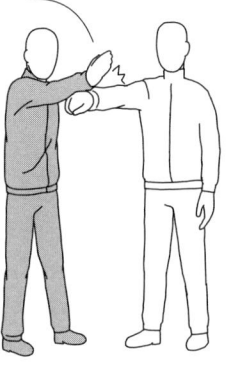

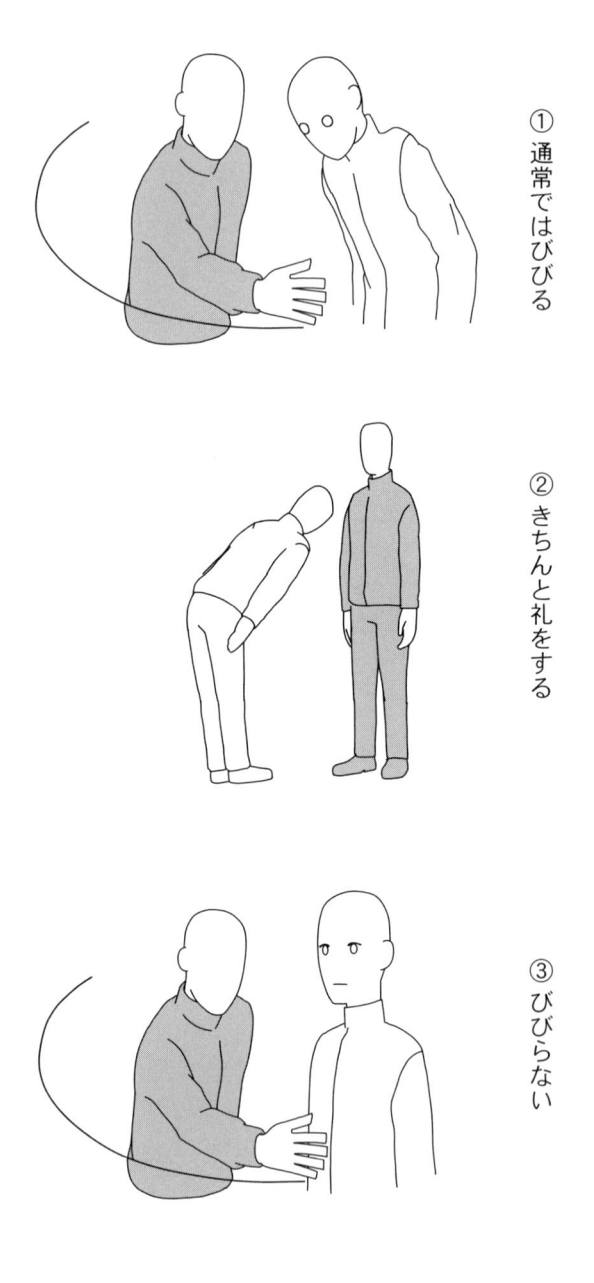

呼吸による身体の [変化C] びびらない

同じく③の時に、今度は腹を平手でいきなり叩くようなふりをしてみます。通常だとそのようにされたらびびりますが、身体に気が通った状態では全くびびることはありません。

① 通常ではびびる

② きちんと礼をする

③ びびらない

このように、身体の呼吸ができると、以上の変化ABCような、「重くなる、強くなる、びびらなくなる」などの変化が一瞬にして起こります。これが身体に気が流れている状態、すなわち「統一体」の状態です。

「統一体」とは、身体をバラバラに捉えた部分体ではなく最初からひとつであると捉えるあり方を言います。身体は心とも関係していて、統一体とは身体のみでなく心と身体も一致している状態です。それは人間はもともと一個の受精卵から細胞分裂を繰り返して37兆個の細胞となる、すなわちスタートからしてひとつの生命体であるからです。

そしてこの身体を構成している37兆個の細胞と細胞の中にある2万4千個のDNAそのものに、「ある条件下に置かれると身体が最適な答えを出す」という能力が最初から備わっているのです。

この例では「きちんとする」ということがその条件にあたりますが、このことで身体と呼吸が一致して気が流れ変化が起きるわけです。

ところが、この検証の時に、いいかげんな礼をしたり、ポケットに手をつっこんだような横着な態度で相手に向き合ったり、「やった！」とガッツポーズをとるような調子にのった態度をとると、とたんに上記のような変化は起こらなくなります。**なぜなら身体の気の**

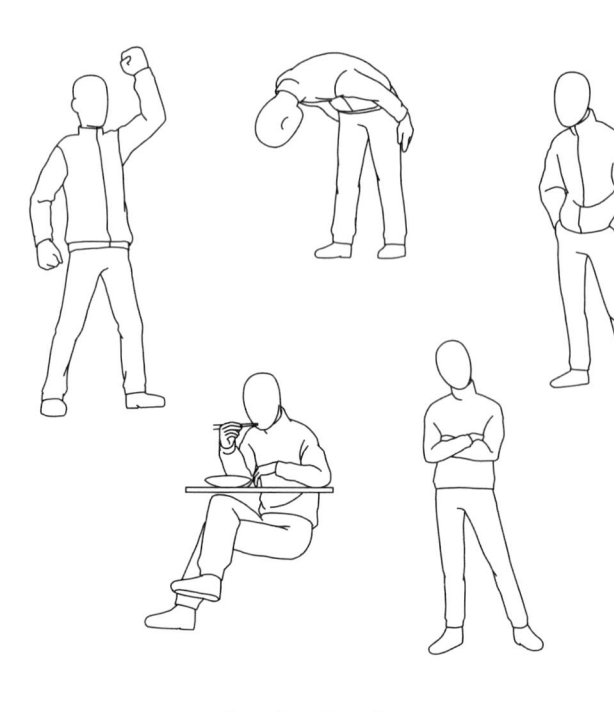

日常には身体の気の流れを止める所作があふれている

流れは心の状態とも深く関係しているからです。このように身体に気が通る所作と気が通らない誤った所作では、一方で人間とは何かという本質も見えてくるのではないかと言えます。

このように身体が身心一致の状態となった時に初めて、本来の力を発揮できる状態となります。本書ではまずは身体の気を止めない、気を流す呼吸法を紹介していきます。

第二章 宇城式呼吸法

—— 統一体をつくる ——

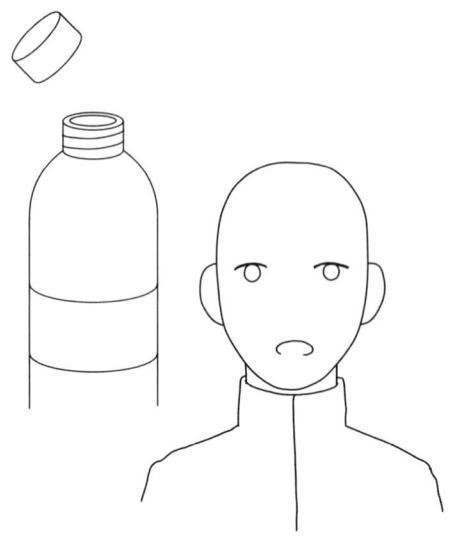

宇城式呼吸法の基本は、まず口を軽くぱっと開けます。

口を開けた時は、息を吸うでもなく、吐くでもなく、ただぱっと口を開けるだけにします。これだけで身体は口を開けない時よりも強くなります。

ペットボトルはフタを取ることによって中の水が自由に出入りできるようになりますが、それは身体でも同じで、ただ口をぱっと開けることで、身体の中に空気が出入りし、身体が自然な状態と

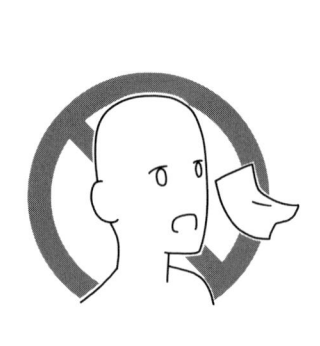
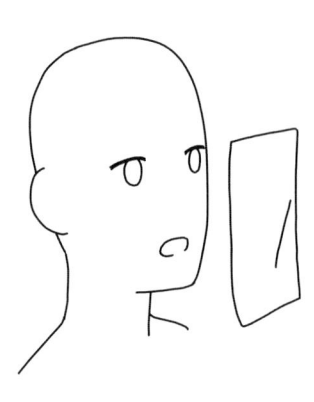

なります。

その上で次に鼻から息を吸い、手の動きに合わせて口でゆっくり吐いていきます。吐く時に重要なことは、息を前方向に吐き出すのではなく、息を身体の中を通して下方へ落としこむように吐いていくということです。

呼吸が正しくできているかどうかを見るには、ティッシュペーパーを口の前に垂らし、そこで息を吐いてみるとわかりやすいと思います。

息を吐いた時にティッシュペーパーが前にゆらいでしまう時は呼吸の空気が前に働いている状態です。それは正しいあり方ではありません。息を吐いてもゆらがない、すなわち息が体内を通って下へ落ちていくことが重要です。正しくできているかどうかは、これで確認してみてください。

① 両手を胸の前に揃える

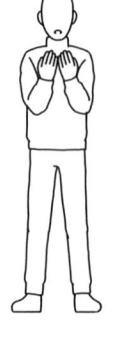

② 前へ

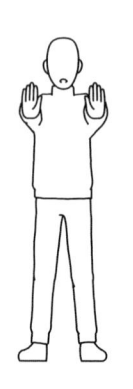

③ 胸の前に戻す

① まず両手を胸の前に揃えます。

② 口をぱっと開け、鼻から少し吸って、そこから呼吸を身体の中を下方に吐きながらゆっくりと両手を前方へまっすぐ伸ばします。肘はおおむね伸ばし手の平は立てて外に向けます。手の動きに合わせて息を吐いていきます。

③ 両手をゆっくり元の胸の位置に戻します。

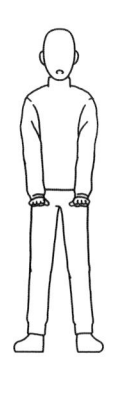

⑥下へ

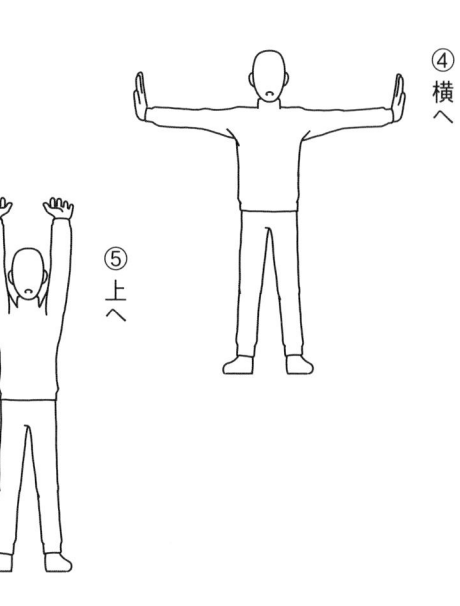

④横へ

⑤上へ

この時、手の平は自分に向きます。手を戻す時の息は、自然体で腹ではなく胸で吸い込むような気持ちで。

④次は真横へゆっくりと伸ばします。手の平は立てます。呼吸は前方の時と同じです。

⑤両手を胸の位置に戻し、次は両手を真上に伸ばします。手の平は上に向け軽く持ち上げるような感じで。

⑥両手を胸の位置に戻し、次は下へ伸ばします。手の平は大地をファーッと押さえていくような気持ちで。両手をゆっくり元の胸の位置に戻します。

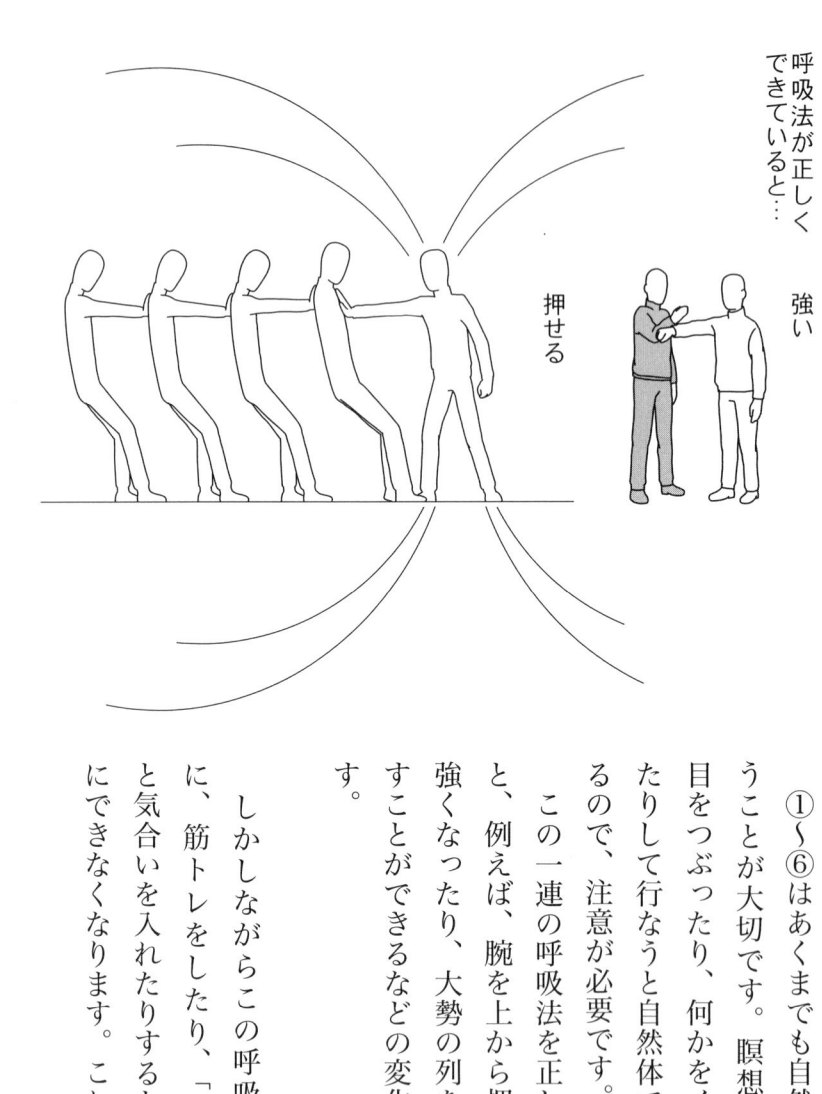

呼吸法が正しく
できていると…

強い

押せる

①〜⑥はあくまでも自然体で行なうことが大切です。瞑想をしたり、目をつぶったり、何かをイメージしたりして行なうと自然体ではなくなるので、注意が必要です。

この一連の呼吸法を正しく行なうと、例えば、腕を上から押さえても強くなったり、大勢の列を簡単に押すことができるなどの変化があります。

しかしながらこの呼吸法のあとに、筋トレをしたり、「よっしゃ」と気合いを入れたりすると、とたんにできなくなります。これは呼吸法

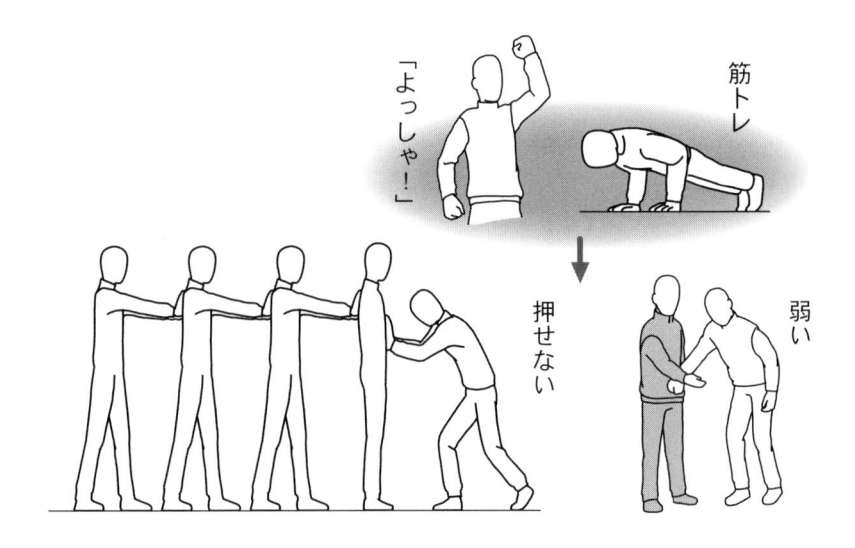

筋トレ

「よっしゃ！」

押せない

弱い

によってせっかく身体に呼吸が通っ
て身体が相手と調和した状態となっ
ていたのを、壊してしまうからです。
すなわち対立の状態に戻ってしまう
からです。

対立の状態となると、孤立状態に
なり、大地とも調和できなくなるの
で、大地のエネルギーを身体に取り
込むことができなくなります。

この対立の要因やその弊害につい
てはのちほど詳しく述べます。

宇城式呼吸法は、身体動作と呼吸の連携を主体とした鍛錬法なので、ノルマ的なエクササイズに陥ると、その効果を失ってしまいます。

そこで道塾ではこの呼吸法をやる時に、以下のような「言葉」を発したあとに動作をするようにしてもらっています。

① 両手を前に出す時、まず「私からあなたへ」と言うか、心の中で思い、感謝をする。

② 両手を横へ出す時は、「私から皆さんへ」と言うか、心の中で思い、感謝を込める。

③ 両手を上に上げる時は、「天に感謝」。

④ 両手を下に下げる時は、「地に感謝」。

この一連の動作を伴った「感謝の型」によって自然に身体に呼吸を通すことができます。

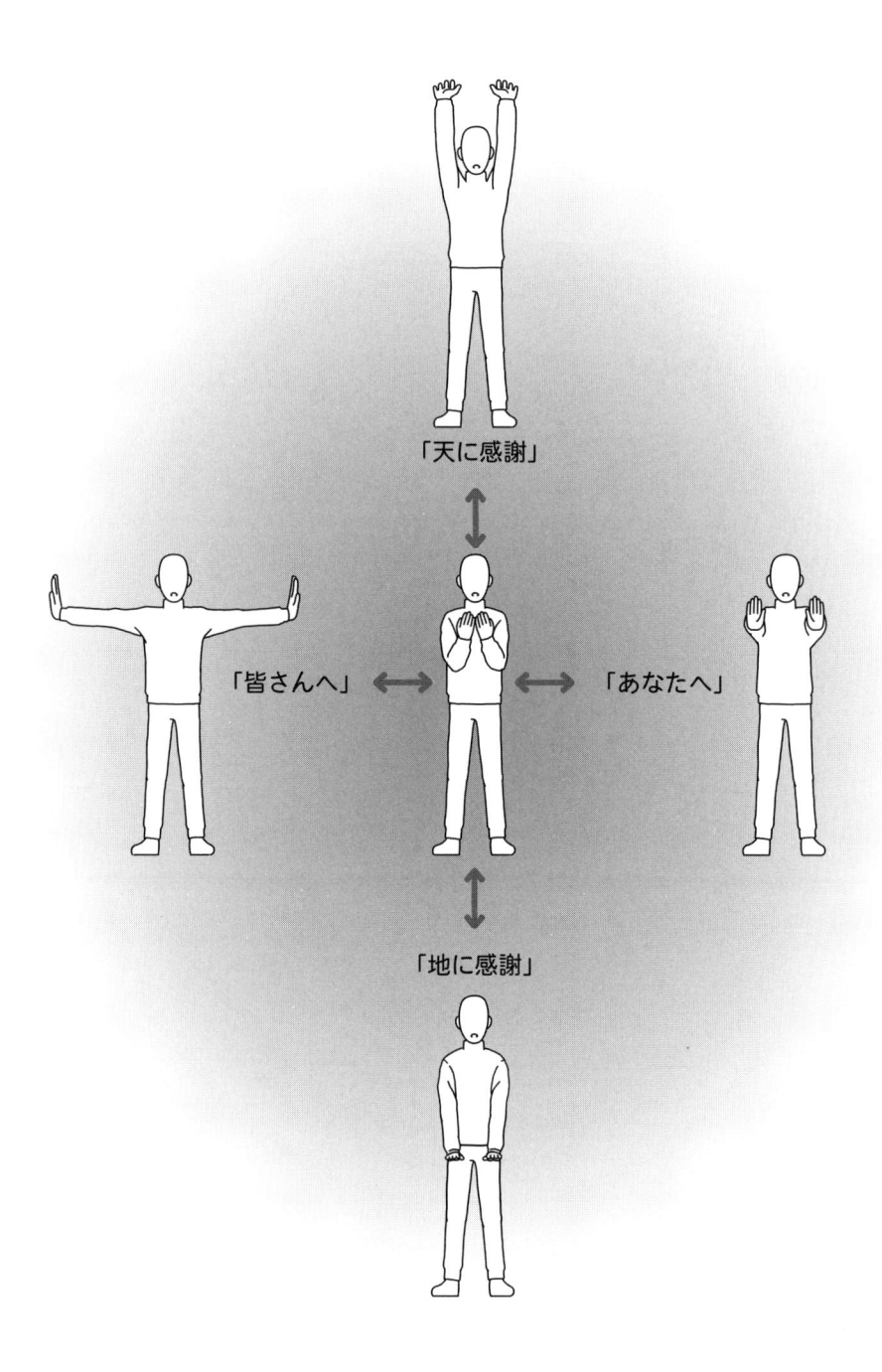

「天に感謝」

「皆さんへ」 ↔ ↔ 「あなたへ」

「地に感謝」

しかしこれも言葉と心が一致してこそ有効であり、感謝の言葉を発したとしても、心と言葉が一致していなければ呼吸は通りません。

例えば両手を前に出す時に、「私からあなたへ」ではなく、「俺から貴様へ」と言いながら行なってみると、身体と呼吸の一致が起こらず、身体は弱くなります。これはやってみれば明白です。検証で呼吸が通っていた時に体感できた「重くなる、強くなる、びびらない」がすべてできなくなります。

これが言葉の力、言霊の持つ力です。

身体は何が正しいかを常に知っていて、間違っていたり、対立したりすると勝手に弱くなり、正しく、調和する状態となると、身体は自然に強くなるのです。

これが身体が知っているという「身体先にありき」という真実です。

昔から日本に伝えられている挨拶の作法や躾として身につけていく正座などの所作に、そうした身体に気が流れる力が隠されているということです。

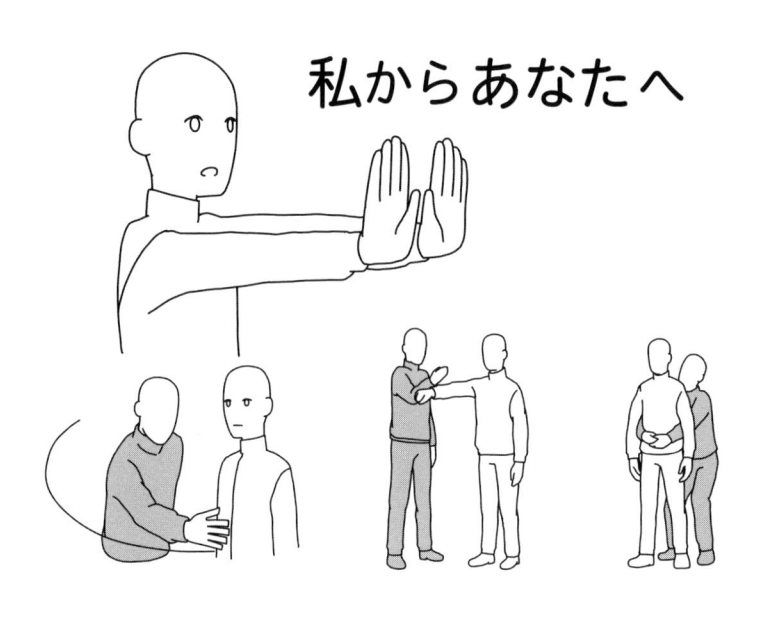

私からあなたへ

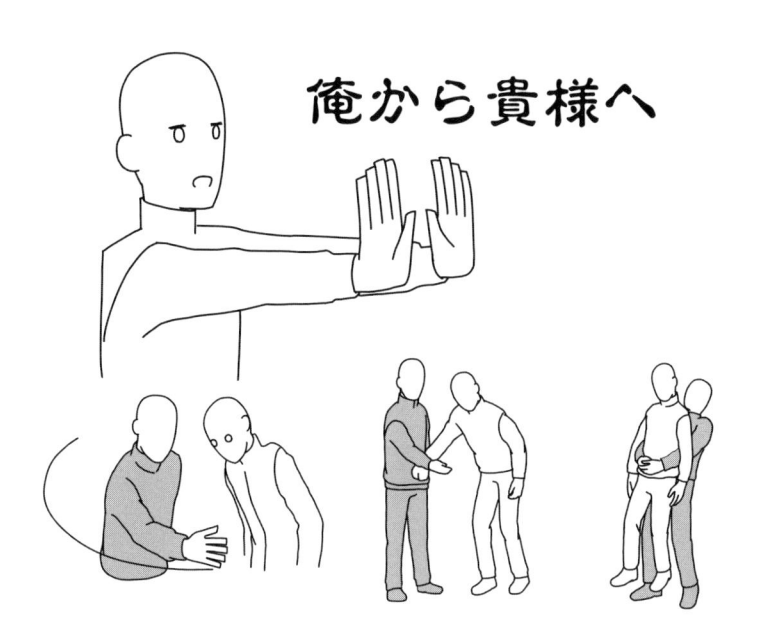

俺から貴様へ

第三章　呼吸法で対立しない身体をつくる

身体の呼吸はなぜ止まるのか

昨今の日本では、身体に呼吸を通らなくし、止めてしまう要因が多々あります。その根底にあるのが「対立」という世界です。

「対立」と言うと、喧嘩や争い、戦争という目に見える形での「衝突」を思い浮べるかと思いますが、実は私たちが日常で「常識」とされていることの中に、たくさんの「対立」「衝突」が潜んでいるのです。

その典型的な例がスポーツや武道に見る試合です。スポーツや武道は一般的にその多くが相対構図をとっています。相対構図というのは衝突であり、対立です。特に最近の傾向は勝つこと、一番になることが主体となり、身体だけでなく心をも対立の状態にさせてしまっています。

相手に勝つことだけに目が向くと、その心は相対的になり対立をつくります。「相手に勝つ」という「相手を相対的に意識した状態」では、身体に呼吸を通すことはできません。この「競う」という「相手を相対的に意識した状態」では、身体に呼吸を通すことはできません。この「競う」という。なぜ

ならば、どんなに「ナンバーワンを目指す」「金メダルを目指す」などというように、美しい言葉で表現したとしても、本質は対立であることは変わりはないからです。対立というように、美しい状態そのものが、身体と心の状態を固まらせ、身体と心の一致を阻害し、気の流れを止めてしまうからです。

筋トレは対立構造をつくる

本来身体を構成している37兆個の細胞は調和構造になっていますが、スポーツなどで勝つために行なわれている筋力トレーニングなどは、逆に対立構造をつくり、身体の呼吸を止める典型的な例と言えます。

それは筋力トレーニングが、もともと生命体として統一体である身体を、わざわざ腕なら腕、足なら足というように、部分体にしてしまうからです。すなわち身体に呼吸が通っている自然体をわざわざ壊してしまうからです。

それは、以下の例のように、自然体の時と、腹筋などの筋トレをした後の身体の状態を比較することで確認することができます。

① 自然体で立って手を前に出す。

② その腕を上から第三者に抑えてもらう。→ **強い**

③ 次に筋トレの腹筋をする。

④ 立ち上がり手を前に出して②と同じように上から押さえてもらう。→ **弱い**

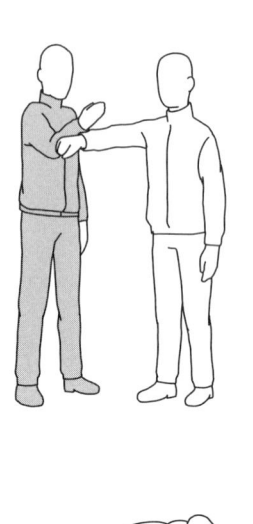

① ② 強い

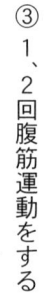

③ 1、2回腹筋運動をする

④ 弱い

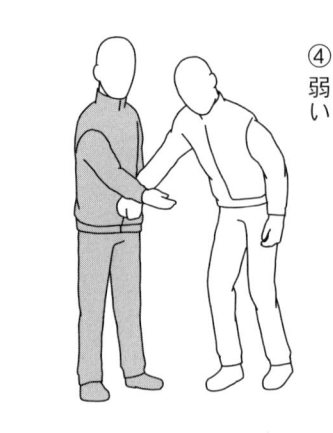

身体が自然体で整っている状態「統一体」では、手を上から押さえられてもその力を身体全体で受け止めることができていました。ところが筋トレをすることによって身体が「部分体」になり、腕と身体全体が切り離されて、全体から生まれる力が発揮できなくなって

しまっています。これが呼吸が詰まっている状態で、身体は大変弱い状態となります。

こうした部分トレーニングのあり方の弊害は、身体的なことのみでなくメンタルな部分でも顕著です。それは以下のような検証を通して気づくことができます。

がんばるぞ（心の対立）で呼吸がつまり、身体の気が止まる

例えば、ガッツポーズをしながら、「がんばるぞ！」と気合いを入れてみます。そして36頁の腹筋運動の時と同じように手を前に出してそれを上から押さえてもらうと、弱くなっているのが分かります。

これは、身体が「頑張れない」ことを知っている状況の時は、いくら言葉で「がんばろう」と言っても、この身体と心の不一致が対立構造をつくり、身体を弱く

① ガッツポーズをする

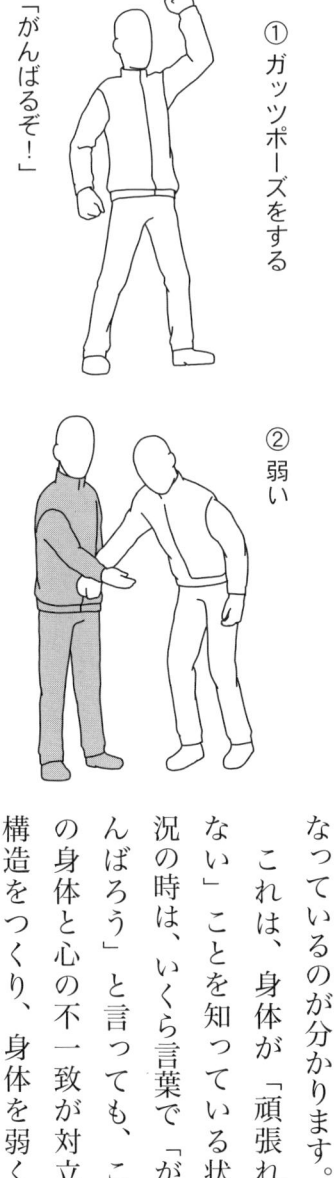

「がんばるぞ！」

② 弱い

してしまうからです。

今の常識に見るトレーニングの筋力アップによる強さへの追究は、それ自体がそもそも対立構造をつくる要因となっているのです。このことへの理解は、頭や理屈ではむずかしいですが、身体を通して体験するとよくわかります。道塾では実際に様々な検証を通して「対立」の事実を体験することで理解を深めていきます。

さらに道塾では、この対立に対し、調和の心があれば身心は一致し、対立を乗り越えることができることも学んでいきます。

大切なことは競うことではなく、自分を高めていくメカニズムを学び、本来人間に備わっている潜在力を発揮できるよう努力をすることです。そのことによって本当の自信を得ることができるのです。

日常に潜む呼吸を止める常識

呼吸を止める常識① 体育座り

身体の呼吸を止め、気の流れを滞らせる要因は日常の生活の中にも多く潜んでいます。

例えば、日本の学校などで子供たちが座って話を聞く時の「体育座り」もその一つです。

なぜこの座り方が身体の呼吸を止めるのかは、正座をした時の比較で分かります。体育座りの時に横から押すと簡単に倒れますが、一方、正座の時は簡単には倒れず強いです。

また、体育座りをしたあとに立ち上がり同じ検証をします（→弱い）。今度は正座をきちんとしてから立ち上がって同じ検証をします（→強い）。これはやってみれば誰もがその違いを確認することができます。（この検証については、『心と体 つよい子に育てる躾』や『人間の潜在力』でも紹介していますので参照してください。）

前述の立礼の検証で、身体を構成している37兆個の細胞と細胞の中にある2万4千個のDNAそのものに、「ある条件下に置かれると身体が最適な答えを出す」という能力が最初から備わっている」ことを述べましたが、正座といういきちんとした座り方こそ、その力を引き出す土台のひとつなのです。これに対し「体育座り」は、それを根底から崩してしまう座り方であるのです。

この「体育座り」は1958年頃から文部省によって学校に取り入れられた座り方と言われ、それ以前

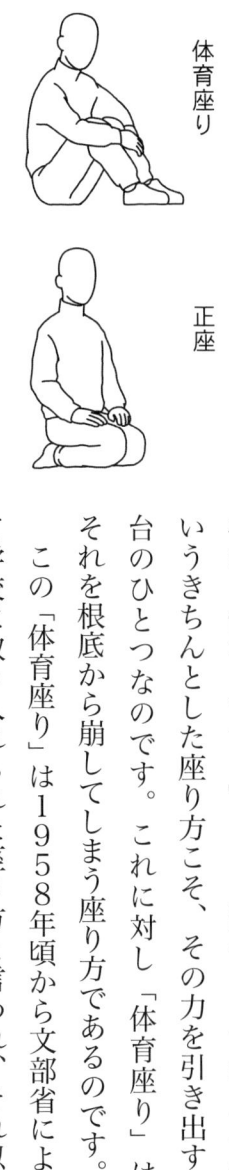

体育座り

正座

に学校に在籍した人は経験のない姿勢であると言います。いわばここ60年の間に急速に日本に広まった座り方であり、しかも、この座り方を導入した理由も、主に子供たちを教師の話に集中させたり、動いたりさせないようにするためだとされ、子供の側に立って考えられた座り方ではありません。（参考　竹内敏晴著　『表現への出発』）。

この体育座りは、それ以降学校教育の場の座り方として定着し、現代に至っているわけですが、これまで一度もこの体育座りのあり方とその弊害が検討されてこなかったことは大変残念であると思います。

検証から明らかなように、この姿勢は瞬時に子供たちの呼吸を止め、したがって身体の気の流れ止め、身体を弱くしてしまいます。集中するどころか、かえって身体の集中を阻害してしまうあり方であるのです。最近の子供は切れやすいとか、集中力がないとか言われていますが、その原因をつくっているのが真に何であるか、今一度、右記のような検証を参考に、改めて検討されるべきではないかと考えます。

呼吸を止める常識②　準備体操（ラジオ体操）

同じく学校現場や広く公の場で行なわれているラジオ体操ですが、この体操は部分の体

一般的な
脇を伸ばす運動

宇城式統一体体操の
脇を伸ばす運動

操としてはよく考えられている体操ではありますが、身体に呼吸を通す「統一体」という観点から見ると大きな課題があります。その事はこれまでの検証例と同じく体験することでその差がより明確になります。

例えば、ラジオ体操の代表的な運動に、身体を横に曲げる運動があります。この運動は、身体を横に曲げることによって脇腹の筋肉を伸ばし消化器官の働きを促進させるとされていますが、この横に曲げた時の姿勢は、横から押されると、とたんに身体が崩れてしまいます。

身体が押されてゆらいでしまうということは、身体に呼吸が通っていない、すなわち気が流れていない状態であるということです。

これを呼吸が通った運動にするには、イラス

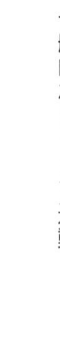

一般的なジャンプ運動

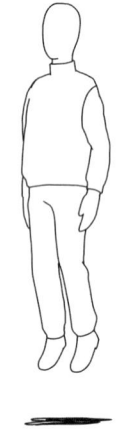

相手を投げることができない

トのように両手の平を向き合わせるようにして横に曲げます。この状態で先ほどと同じように横から押します。先ほどのラジオ体操と違って強くなり、ぐらつくことはありません。どんな運動も、この例のように身体に呼吸が通っていることが大切であるのです。気を通す体操こそ身体を強くする形になるからです。

もう一つのラジオ体操の典型的な例に、両足をそろえてジャンプする運動があります。これは脚部の筋肉を活発に動かすことで全身の血行をよくし体の緊張をほぐす運動とされていますが、実際そうなっているのか、それはこの運動後に身体がどういう状態になっているかを検証することで、その大きな課題に気づくことができます。

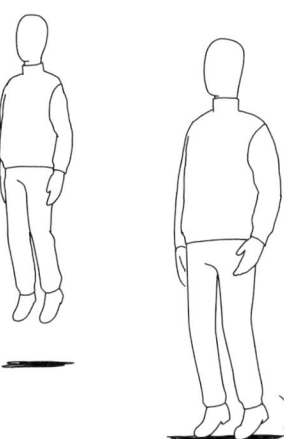

宇城式統一体体操のジャンプ運動

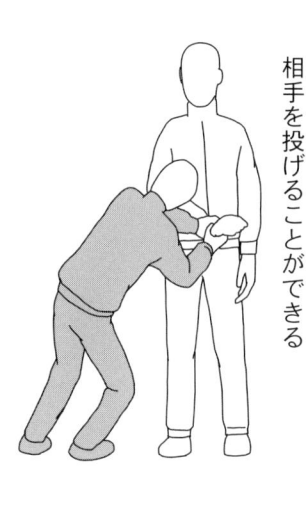

相手を投げることができる

　まず通常のラジオ体操のように両足をそろえてジャンプをします。

　そのあとの身体の変化を確認する一つの方法として、腕をしっかりつかんでもらいます。そのまま相手を投げようとしても、投げることができません。

　これに対し、宇城式統一体体操のジャンプは、まずつま先を地面に付けたままジャンプを開始し、数回そうしたあとにふつうにジャンプをします。

　このあとに先ほどと同じように、相手に腕をつかんでもらいます。今回はびっくりするほど力が出て相手を倒すことができます。

なぜこういう差異が起こるのか。それはラジオ体操や筋力トレーニングは部分強化しての効果はあるものの、生命体本来の力を出すことにはつながっていないからです。**生命体**としての力を発揮するには気の通った統一体になることが必要です。

先ほどのラジオ体操の、上体を横に倒す運動やジャンプの運動はまさに身体を破壊し、部分体とする運動です。それを宇城式統一体体操をすることによって身体を元の状態に戻すことができるので、再び強くなるということです。ですから宇城式統一体体操を「復活体操」とも呼んでいます。

呼吸を止める常識③ 心なし（心ありが呼吸をつくる）

身体に呼吸が通るか通らないかは、心のあり方でも大きく影響を受けます。他人を思いやる「心あり」の状態か、自分さえよければという孤立した「心なし」の状態とでは身体の呼吸も重みも大きく異なってきます。

例えば、道端に具合が悪そうにしている人がいて、この時に、自分には関係ないと見て見ぬふりをして通り過ぎたとします。この時にその通り過ぎた人を後ろから抱き上げると、不思議なほど軽々と持ち上がってしまいます。

ところが、その同じ人が今度は具合が悪そうな人のほうへ歩み寄って、「どうしたんですか」と声をかけてみると、その人を同じように抱き上げても、先ほどよりもずっと重くなっているのが分かると思います。

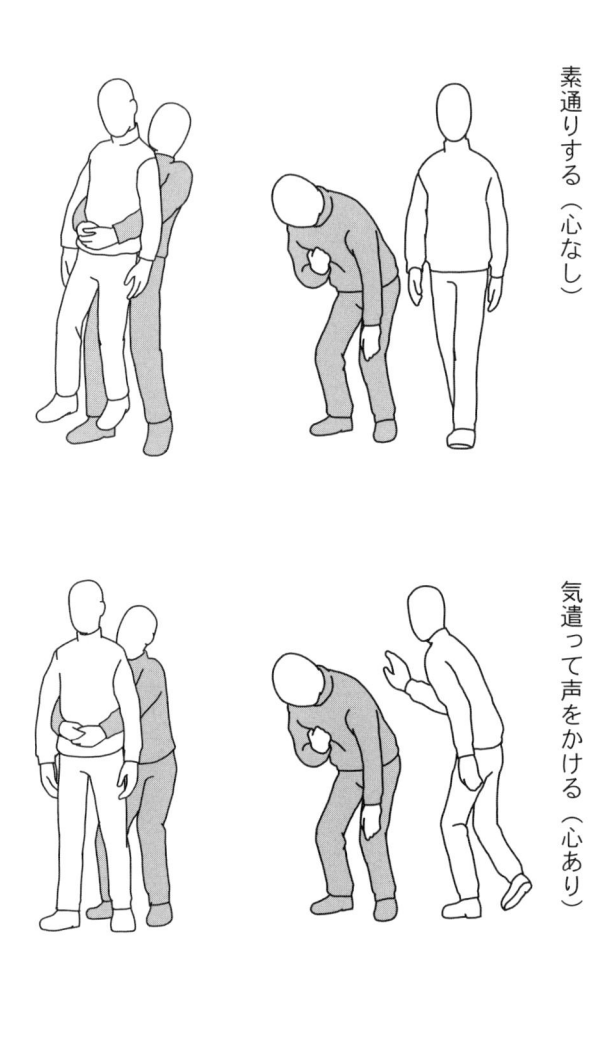

素通りする（心なし）

気遣って声をかける（心あり）

「心なし」だと身体の呼吸が止まって身体が軽くなり、「心あり」だと身体の呼吸が自然にでき、気が流れるので身体が重くなるのです。

これは実際にやってみると違いが明白であり、いかに目に見えない心の状態が身体に影響を与えるものか、分かりやすい例と言えるでしょう。

このように心のあり方で**身体は軽くも重くもなり、外からは見えなくても身体は常に答えを出している**ということです。

すなわち身体に呼吸が通り気が流れ、相手やまわりと調和することができれば、身体は重くかつゆらぐことなく、統一体となり、本来の力を発揮できる状態となるのです。

身体の呼吸ができていて身体の各部がすべて全体につながっている状態が統一体です。

身体に気が通ったこの統一体の状態であれば、怪我や疲れも少なくなります。

現在スポーツで行なわれている西洋式の準備体操やラジオ体操は、部分の筋力パワーアップや柔軟性を主体とするもので、身体全体を自然体に強くするものではありません。

真の体操とは、部分に働きかけるものではなく、身体全体の細胞に働きかけるものでなく

てはなりません。

宇城式統一体体操は、身体全体を整え気を通す身体操法です。

この統一体体操は、『気の開発メソッド　初級編』で詳しく紹介していますので参照してください。

本来の身体の呼吸を取り戻す

宇城式呼吸法はこのように、腹式とか胸式とか丹田など、身体の各部を「意識して」鍛えたりエクササイズとして行なう部分体的プログラムではなく、あくまでも身体を自然体という統一体に戻し、生命体としての本来の力を発揮させるベースをつくる呼吸法です。

まずは、呼吸が通った身体、すなわち気が通った身体であるかどうかの違いを自分自身で体感し、本来の身体を自分の中に取り戻す方向へ向かうことが大切です。

自然体の身体となれば、身体は居付いたりこわばったりせずに自由な動きが可能となります。バラバラだった身体が一つになり、気が流れ始めます。

そして、気が流れている身体とそうでない身体の違いに気づくことができます。

「ああ、これが自然体の身体なのだ」と理解できた時がその第一歩です。

そうした本来の自然体の身体を取り戻すことこそ自らに眠るエネルギーを引き出すベースとなります。

そしてそれは武術の極意にも通じる、隙のない身体をつくる呼吸法とも言えます。

本書を通し、多くの方が本来の身体の呼吸を取り戻すきっかけになることを願っています。

本書の参考としての動画です。QRコードまたはURLでアクセスし、パスワードを入力してご覧ください。

**宇城式呼吸法
および 検証方法**

Pass: usb005j

https://www.dou-shuppan.com/movie_kokyuho/

宇城憲治 うしろけんじ

1949 年 宮崎県小林市生まれ。1986 年 由村電器㈱ 技術研究所所長、1991 年 同常務取締役、1996 年 東軽電工㈱ 代表取締役、1997 年 加賀コンポーネント㈱ 代表取締役。エレクトロニクス分野の技術者として、ビデオ機器はじめ衛星携帯電話などの電源や数々の新技術開発に携わり、数多くの特許を取得。また、経営者としても国内外のビジネス界第一線で活躍。一方で、厳しい武道修行に専念し、まさに文武両道の日々を送る。
現在は徹底した文武両道の生き様と武術の究極「気」によって人々の潜在能力を開発する指導に専念。宇城空手塾、宇城塾、教師塾、各企業・学校講演、プロ・アマ スポーツ塾などで、「学ぶ・教える」から「気づく・気づかせる」の指導を展開中。著書・DVD 多数。

㈱ＵＫ実践塾 代表取締役	創心館空手道 範士九段
宇城塾総本部道場 創心館館長	全剣連居合道 教士七段（無双直伝英信流）
宇城道塾塾長	

ＵＫ実践塾ホームページ　http://www.uk-jj.com

宇城道塾

東京・大阪・仙台・名古屋・岡山・熊本で開催。随時入塾を受け付けています。
　宇城道塾ホームページ　http://www.dou-shuppan.com/dou
　事務局　TEL: 042-766-1117　Email: do-juku@dou-shuppan.com

公式テキスト：『気の開発メソッド　初級編／中級編』 季刊『道（どう）』
教材ＤＶＤ：『宇城空手 in Aiki Expo』『永遠なる宇城空手』
　　　　　　『宇城憲治　ネパール・ムスタン訪問記録』

宇城道塾の手引き　〈実践編①〉
身体に気を流す 宇城式呼吸法

2019 年 6 月 26 日　初版第 1 刷発行
2022 年 3 月 1 日　　　第 2 刷発行

宇城道塾事務局編　宇城憲治監修

定　価　本体価格 1,400 円
発行者　渕上郁子
発行所　株式会社 どう出版
　　　　〒 252-0313　神奈川県相模原市南区松が枝町 14-17-103
　　　　電話 042-748-2423（営業）　042-748-1240（編集）
　　　　http://www.dou-shuppan.com
印刷所　株式会社シナノパブリッシングプレス

© Kenji Ushiro 2019　Printed in Japan　ISBN978-4-910001-00-5
落丁、乱丁本はお取り替えいたします。お読みになった感想をお寄せください。

Ushiro Dou Juku Handbook

Practical Application 1

Compiled and drafted by the Editorial Board of Dou Juku
Supervised by Kenji Ushiro

Ushiro-Style Breathing

Streaming Ki through the Body

About the Author,
Kenji Ushiro

Kenji Ushiro is a business executive, engineer and martial arts expert. He has been involved in developing new technology for numerous electronic devices, ranging from video equipment to satellite cell phones, and has been granted many patents.

In addition, he has devoted himself to intense martial arts training and led a life of true "bunbu ryodo" – the unified path of martial arts and everday life.

Born in 1949, Mr. Ushiro is the 9th Dan Hanshi of Soshinkan Karatedo and a 7th Dan Kyoshi in Iaido within the All-Japan Kendo Federation. He was Head of the Technological Research Institute of Yoshimura Electric Company, Ltd. and became Managing Director in 1986. He became President of Kaga Components Company, Ltd. in 1997.

In 2004, he founded his own Karate school, UK Jissen Juku. Since retiring from the corporate world, he has devoted himself to teaching not only Karate students but people from all walks of life and backgrounds including professional athletes, coaches, university and high school students and business executives. The age of his students range from 6 to 75. He teaches within and outside Japan using his revolutionary instructional method, Ki.

(c)2019 by Kenji Ushiro

Translated by
Josh Drachman

Published by Dou Shuppan
Phone: 042-748-1240 E-mail: shop@dou-shuppan.com
#103, 14-17 Matsugae-cho Minami-ku Sagamihara-shi
Kanagawa-ken, 252-0313 Japan
http://www.dou-shuppan.com/

Printed in Japan   ISBN 978-4-910001-00-5

Introduction

What Our Natural Bodies Should Be Like

In the basic version of the Dou Juku Handbook, we have introduced the fundamental concepts and knowledge base of Ushiro Sensei's outlook, thinking, and way of living.

There we brought forward the basic practical program for actualizing the Human Potential we are born with naturally. One part of this program is Ushiro-style breathing.

Ushiro-style breathing is a training method that establishes a return to the body's original state and is purposed for using the body freely, without getting stuck or impeded in any way. It is not a how-to regime of exercises for doing this or that to make ki flow.

It is best to think of it as a program that causes one to realize that constant ki flow and body breathing is our natural original condition.

The Shift in Learning from "Teach and Study" to "Becoming and Being Made Aware"

Learning at Dou Juku is entirely about becoming aware of everything from direct experience through one's own body. The typical style of learning at school and seminars is for the teacher to teach and the student to learn. It goes in one direction and results in students acquiring knowledge with their heads. But at Dou Juku the emphasis is on actively understanding using one's own body.

The theory and practice developed in this series is based on

the actual implementation and fact that verifiable proof lies in what is ahead. According to Ushiro Sensei, the literature and analysis of current science is full of contradictions from the perspective of "proof lies in what is ahead."

In the classes conducted at Dou Juku, scientific theory and writings are actually validated putting contradictions and logic of science in stark contrast with the accumulation of actual proofs.

As Ushiro Sensei says, humans are not like airplanes, cars or personal computers which can be constructed from parts using a blue print. Humans cannot be made from any kind of science or collection of Nobel Prize winners. All that can be said is humans are a mysterious creation of the universe.

Returning to oneself inside is the actual enablement of our extraordinary latent capacity contained in the mystery of humanness — this is the importance of what is taught at Dou Juku. This enablement is not imparted to the body through knowledge-based learning.

One has to recognize that one's own body has been able to do the impossible, even despite one's head saying that these actions cannot be done. This ties into the next step, awareness, which becomes the driving force for study.

The opportunity for this awareness, freed from the blinders of logic, is the actual enablement offered at Dou Juku. It is our hope that the "The Way of Breathing" will help provide a variety of such insights and awareness.

The Staff of Dou Juku

Contents

Chapter 1:

The Meaning of Breathing

The Meaning of Breathing

Breathing, as it is referred to herein and throughout Dou Juku documentation, is not the ordinary breathing through the mouth and nose but rather body breathing. Breathing in and out through the nose and mouth is vitally important for living beings. There is no substitute for this unconscious breathing during sleep.

There are a number of conscious breathing methods and the one taught at Dou Juku is qualitatively distinct. The students of Dou Juku each directly experience a power and bodily action outside of ordinary consciousness that comes from their individual study of Ki. Ushiro-style breathing becomes their individual base for developing this power and is connected to the inner secrets of martial arts. Freezing up, getting tight, becoming stuck and light in a self defense martial situation-- each has a direct connection to mortal danger. The condition of stopped breathing, whereby the body becomes stuck, tight, and floats is partial body. In the partial body condition, there are openings beyond the areas where consciousness is directed and one is highly unprotected in the surrounding environment. In a martial sense, one can easily be killed.

The Ushiro-style breathing that this book will introduce is a

breathing that creates a body that can protect itself as a unified body that cannot be killed as well as a breathing that gives rise to energy within oneself.

The Harmful Effects in Daily Life of the Body Getting Stuck

One may not realize the body's freezing up or the stoppage of breathe, but it happens quite frequently in everyday life. The lack of protection and bodily freedom that comes from this body's stoppage of breathing and freezing up brings about a variety of harmful effects in one's everyday life. The advent of surprise, shock, pressure, or haste leads one to feel unstable, stuck and without body breathing. From a martial perspective, the body is left with openings. An accident occurring under these conditions could lead to severe injury. In sports, it is connected to injury; at work, it leads to mistakes and poor results; in human relationships, it makes for trouble and conflict.

To be able to protect oneself and attain one's natural bodily power, it is essential to become free from conscious will and achieve a natural body that is not stuck. And it is important to have ki running through the body. Ki flowing in the body is the body's natural strong and flexible condition. Just as plants grow by taking up nutrients from the earth, so too does the connection humans have to the earth enable a transmission of the energy we receive.

Changes in the Body from Breathing

Through direct experience of the body when ki is flowing and when ki is not flowing, one can well understand the difference between these two conditions. It is necessary to understand through experience the difference between these two states.

The condition of stopped body breathing is not simply one where breath has stopped flowing in and out of the nose and mouth. Rather, for instance, during an arm wrestling match, it is the moment when one uses power to down the opponent, and the body gets stiff. This condition is a stoppage of breathing and ki. As a result, the body tightens, freezes up and becomes fragile. The proof of this is that if the stomach or back are hit when in this condition, one would experience severe pain. One can clearly experience this through a validation of this circumstance.

Changes in the Body through Breathing: Becoming Heavier

1. Two people pair up. One can easily lift up the other from behind. The same result happens even if the person being lifted thinks to make himself heavy.

2. This time, the person being lifted first faces the person lifting and greets him with a proper bow. The result is that the person cannot be lifted and is much heavier.

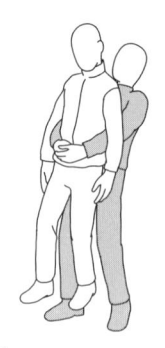 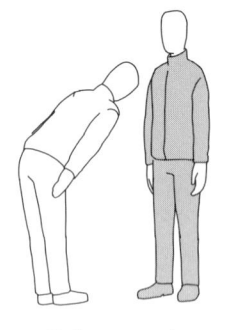 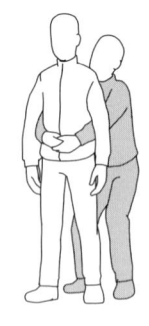

1. The person can be lifted.

2. A proper bow is given.

3. The person cannot be lifted.

Changes in the Body through Breathing: Becoming Stronger

Just as in the last example, the person lifted after giving a proper bow is not only heavy but can now easily throw the person grabbing him. And that person does not feel much pain when his arm is struck as in the diagram. Rather, the person striking feels most of the pain from the attack.

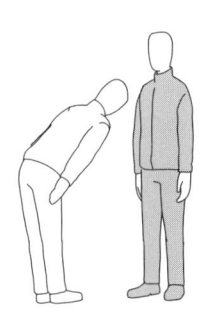 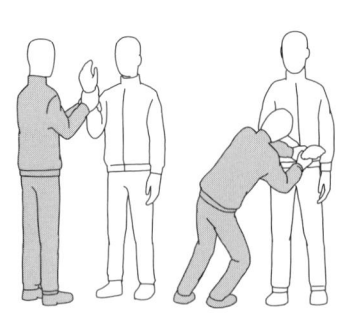 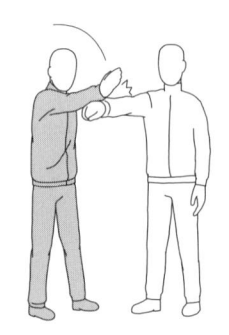

2. A proper bow is given

3-1. The arm is grabbed

3-2. Let the other person fully hit the arm

Change in the Body through Breathing: Not flinching

In this case, the person bows and receives a fake hit to the stomach. Normally such a hit, even a fake one, would cause the person to flinch. But because ki is flowing, he does not flinch at all.

In this way, we can see that once the body can breathe, changes such as becoming stronger, heavier and not flinching instantly occur. This is the condition of ki flow in the body, also known as the "whole body" condition. "Whole body" means the body is not separated or segmented but is, from the outset, one and unified. The body is connected to the heart and in the "whole body" condition, the body and

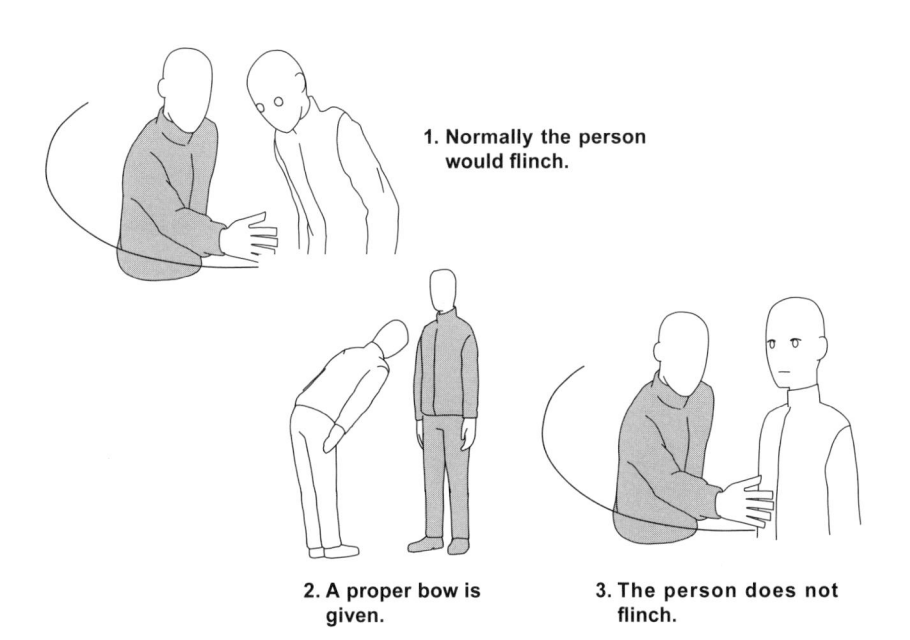

1. Normally the person would flinch.

2. A proper bow is given.

3. The person does not flinch.

heart are one. Humans are, from the start, united living beings that from the repeated subdivision of one fertilized egg eventually become a unified whole of 37 trillion cells.

And from the outset, we are furnished, within the structure of these 37 trillion cells, and the 24,000 DNA strands within each of these cells, with the capacity to set the right conditions to bring out the body's optimal response.

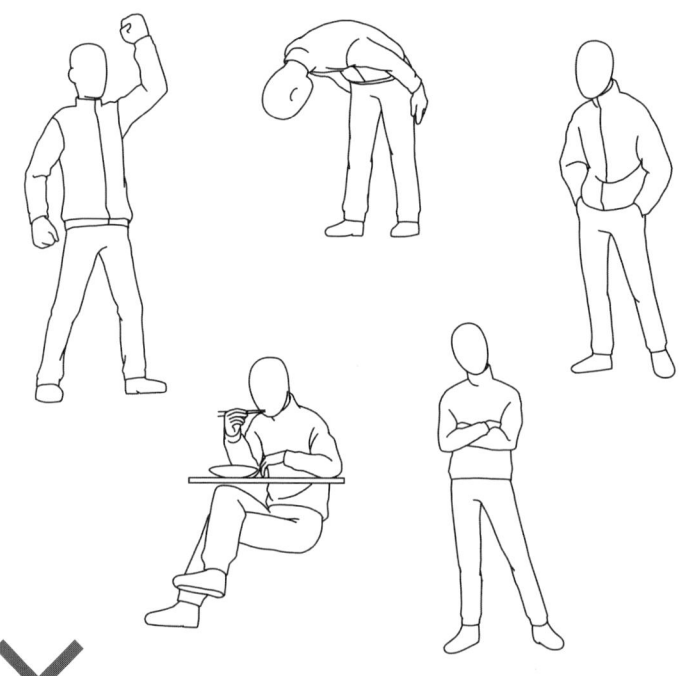

Daily life is full of postures and actions that stop Ki flow

And these conditions will be fulfilled when things are done properly. As a result, body and breathing unite, ki flows and change occurs. But if these conditions are not fulfilled, as, for instance, in the case where one does a sloppy bow or shows an arrogant attitude when doing the validations described above, then the body will not change.

The reason these conditions are fulfilled with proper execution of an action is that the body's ki flow and the condition of the heart are strongly connected. In this way, one's carriage when ki is flowing and not flowing shows a lot about the true nature of human beings.

In this way, when the body is in the condition of mind-body unity, it is the first time we can grasp our true power. Thus, we would like through this book to introduce the way of breathing where the body's ki flows and is not stopped.

Chapter Two:

Creating The Whole Body through Ushiro-Style Breathing

Opening the Mouth Making the Sound "Pah"

In the basics of Ushiro-style breathing, one lightly opens one's mouth making the sound "pah". When one opens the mouth, it is not to breathe in or out but to simply to open making the sound "pah". Simply opening the mouth in this way makes the body stronger than it was when the mouth is closed.

Just as water in a bottle is able to flow in and out freely when the cap is removed, so the air within the body is able to move freely when the mouth is opened. As such, the body's natural condition is restored.

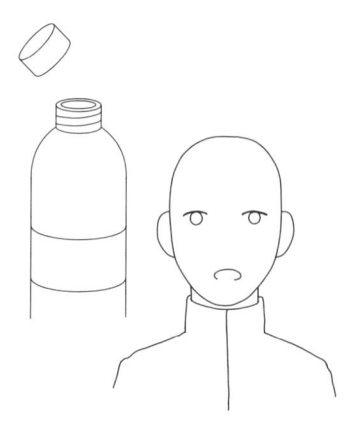

Breathe in through the nose and slowly breathe out in harmony with the movement of your hand. The important thing is that you direct your exhale down and through the inside of your body and not out in the same direction as the inhale. You can easily check if the breathing is correct by placing a piece

of tissue in front of your mouth. If the tissue paper moves, it means the breath is going out and a sign the breathing is not correct. It is important that the tissue paper does not move and that the breath is directed down through the body. You can check the correctness of your breathing using this test.

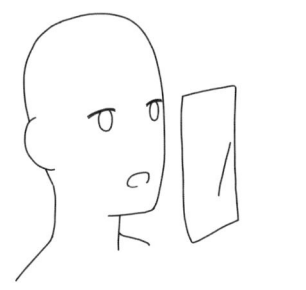 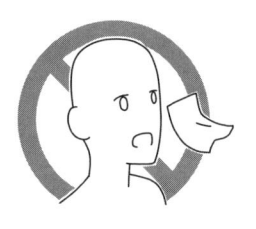

Ushiro-Style Breathing Method

1) First, place both hands in front of your chest.
2) Open your mouth making the "pah" sound. Make a slight breath in through your nose and, then, while directing the exhale down through the inside of the body, extend both hands out straight in front of the body. The elbows are fully extended and the palms are up and facing out. Breathe out in harmony with the movement of the hands.
3) Bring the hands back to their original position in front of the chest and with the palms facing in toward yourself. Use the feeling of the chest drawing in to bring the hands back in, not the hara.
4) Next, slowly stretch the arms to the side with the palms facing up and out with the elbows fully extended;

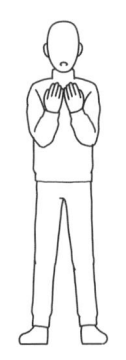

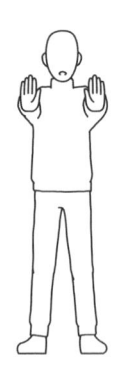

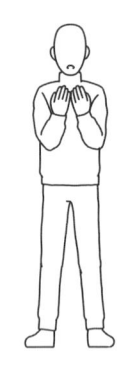

1) Draw both hands to the center of the chest

2) extend them out

3) draw them back to the chest

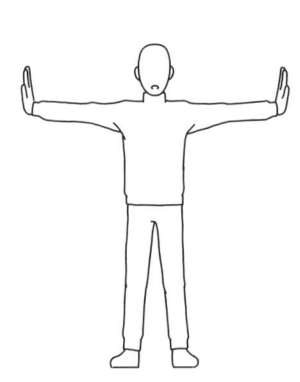

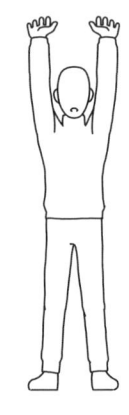

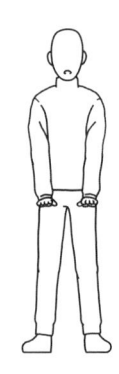

4) extend them to the side and draw them back

5) extend them up and draw them back

6) extend them down, draw them back, repeat the process.

5) bring the arms back in again in front of the chest and then raise them straight up with the feeling of a light stretch with the palms facing upward.

6) Finally, again bring the hands back to the position in front of the chest and extend them downward with the feeling of the hands softly pushing the ground. Then, return the hands to the original position in front of the chest.

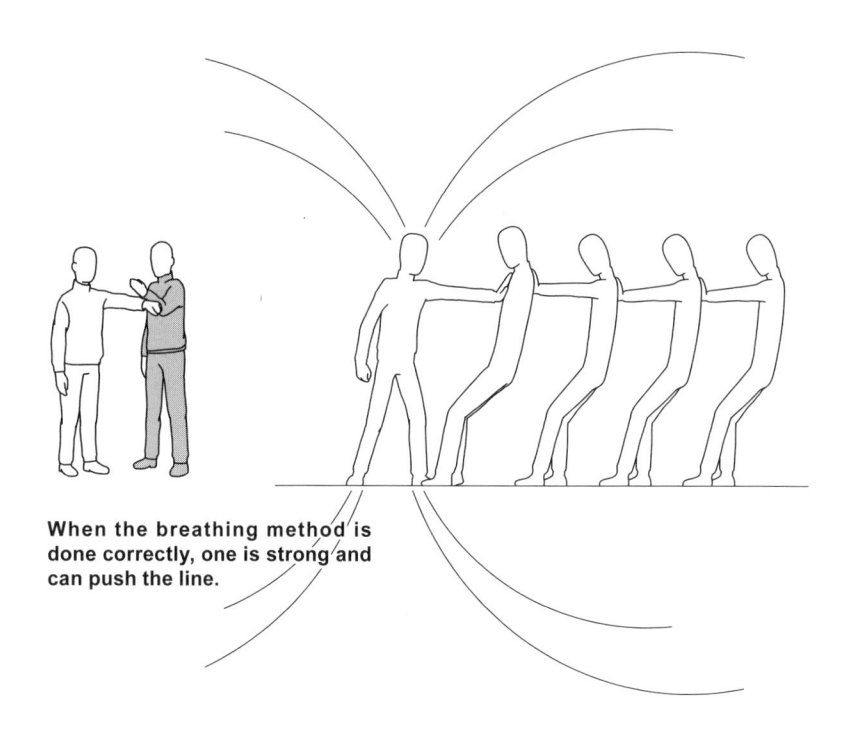

When the breathing method is
done correctly, one is strong and
can push the line.

If one then engages in muscle training or mental motivation saying to oneself, "here we go" or "let's do this!", then one will become weak and cannot move the line.

It is important to be in the natural body condition when doing these six movements. One needs to be aware that closing one's eyes, internal meditation or anything done to create a mental image will not be natural body. Doing this series of breathing movements properly enables changes such as being strong when one's arm is pushed from above and the ability to easily move a long line of people.

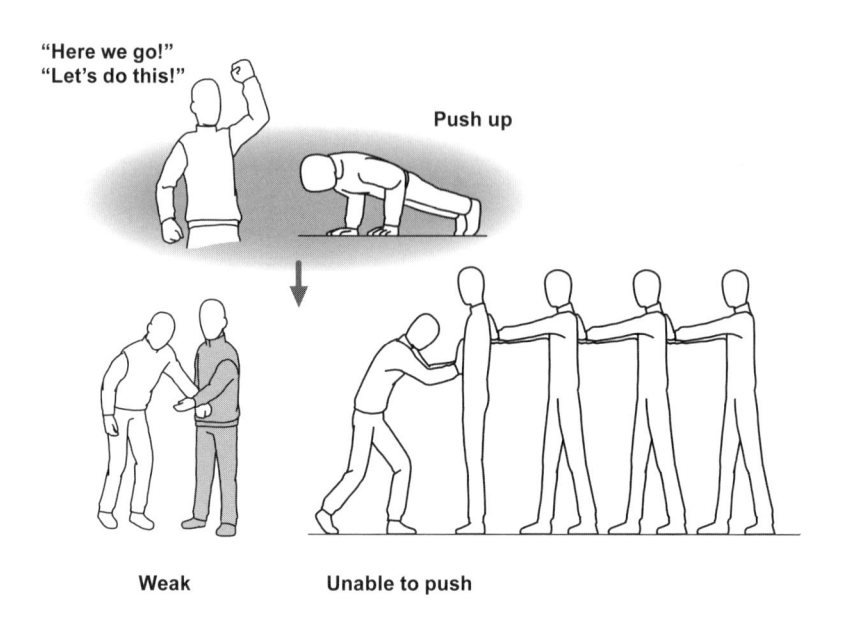

"Here we go!"
"Let's do this!"

Push up

Weak

Unable to push

However, if after doing these breathing exercises, one were to weight lift or engage in a form of willful, self-driven action, then these abilities would instantly go away. These activities would, in effect, destroy the harmonizing and body breathing condition brought about by the breathing method. The body would return to its oppositional state. This oppositional condition leads to isolation and disharmony with the earth and makes it impossible for the body to take in the earth's energy. The origins of this isolation and its negative effects will be discussed in detail later on.

Ushiro-style Breathing Method: The Gratitude Kata Me to You, Me to Everyone, Thanks to the Universe, and Thanks to Earth

Ushiro-style breathing is a training development method that links breathing to body movement. If it is treated as mere exercise, the effect will be lost.

At Dou Juku, we do the breathing exercises and say the following before each movement:

1. Before extending the hands forward, we say "from me to you";
2. Before extending the hands to the side, we say "from me to everyone";
3. Before extending the hands above, we say "thanks to the universe";
4. And, before extending the hands downward, we say "thanks to the earth".

By doing the gratitude kata in this way, breath naturally comes to flow through the body.

Here, too, there is an effect if word and heart are unified. So, if the words of the Gratitude Kata are spoken, but they are not unified with the heart, then the breathing will not flow. For instance, if instead of "from me to you" one were to say "from me to you" without authenticity or respect to the other person, then the body and breath will not unify and the body will become weak. This will become clear if

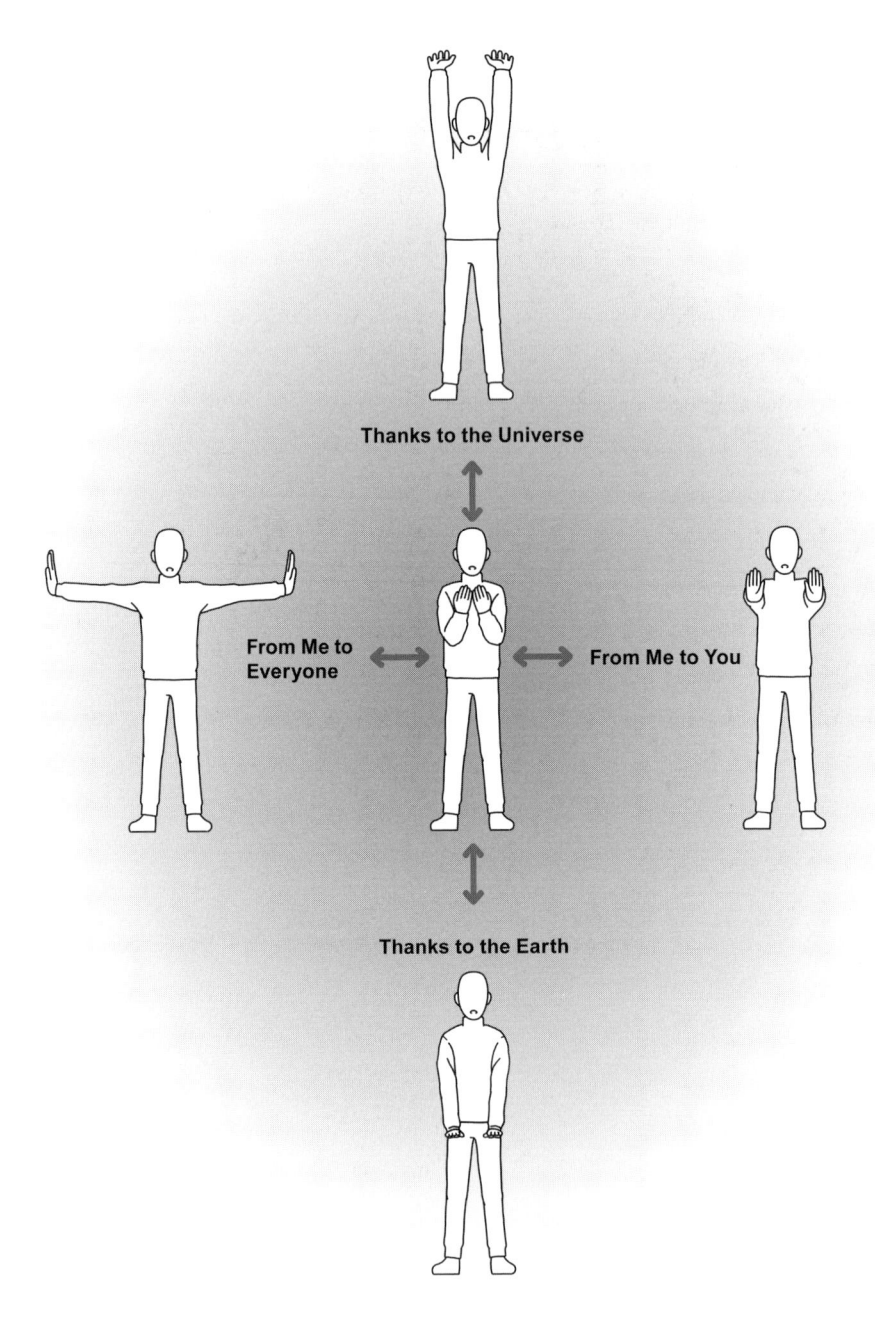

Thanks to the Universe

From Me to Everyone ⟷ ⟷ **From Me to You**

Thanks to the Earth

you try it out. The heaviness, strength, and stability experienced when breath was flowing in the body will all cease to function. This power of the word is known as Kotodama, or "word spirit" in Japanese.

The body always knows whether or not something is correct. When something is wrong or there is conflict, the body naturally becomes weak on its own. When things are correct, the body becomes strong of its own accord. This knowing of when things are right or not right shows the truth that the body is ahead.

The comportment derived from the time-honored Japanese etiquette of proper greeting, sitting seiza and other deeply ingrained manners makes for a body with the hidden power of ki flowing within.

From me to you

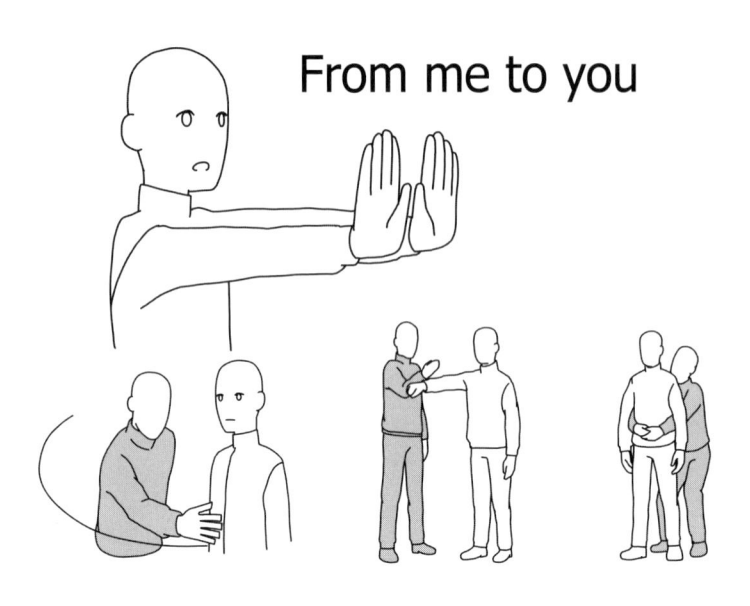

From me to you done without authenticity or respect to the other person

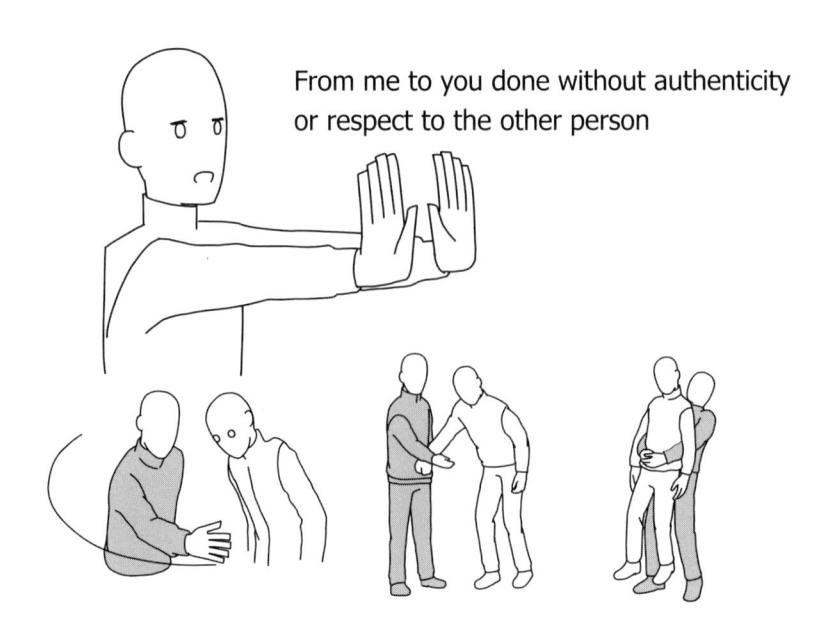

Chapter 3

Using Breathing to Create a Body that Does Not Oppose

Why Does Body Breathing Stop?

There are many reasons why people's body breathing stops and does not flow. The root cause of these is the world of opposition prevalent in modern Japan. The word opposition brings to mind war, battles, fighting and similar visible forms. But, in reality, there many hidden forms of conflict and opposition in the consciousness of our everyday existence.

Competitions in sports and Budo tournaments are typical examples of this conflict. These activities generally have a relativistic structure. And this relativism is inherently oppositional and based on conflict. The modern day emphasis on winning as the main goal changes the condition of the mind and body to opposition. This opposition is created when one sets oneself on beating an opponent, thus producing a confrontational heart.

And because one has a relativistic consciousness of an opponent in competition, breath cannot flow through the body. No matter how beautifully we express the ideals of winning using phrase like "aiming for number one" or "going for the gold", these ideas are, in the end, inherently oppositional in nature. And, as such, the body and mind

become stiff and unable to unify and ki ceases to flow.

Muscle Training Creates the Structure of Opposition

The natural organization of the body, and the 37 trillion cells of which it is comprised, is harmonious. However, the muscle conditioning done in the name of sports competition and winning creates an oppositional structuring which stops body breathing. Muscle training takes our vital, whole-body natural state and purposely turns it into partial body, where an arm is an arm, a leg is a leg without wholistic connection. It purposely destroys the body breathing of the natural body. In the examples below, validations can be made of the natural body compared to that of the body after doing sit ups and other forms of muscle training.

1. In natural stance, one extends the arm.
2. The person is strong when pushed by another person.
3. Then one does a sit up as muscle training.
4. The person re-extends his arm and is weak as the arm can be pushed down by the other person.

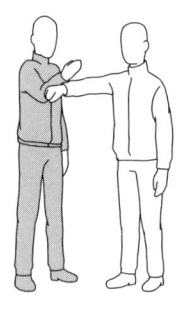 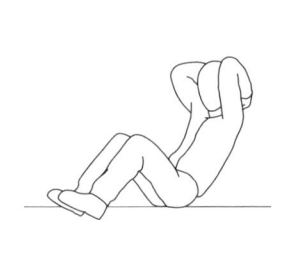 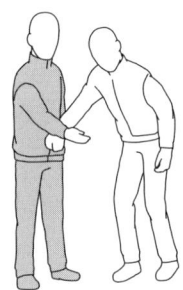

1. 2. One is strong   **3. Repeat steps 1 and 2 after doing sit ups.**   **4. One is weak**

When the body establishes its natural condition as "whole body", the power of the arm pushing down can be received throughout the entire body. However, the partial body induced by muscle training makes the extended arm separate and cut off from the body's entirety and the power it produces. The body breathing gets stopped up and the body gets very weak. The negative effects of this kind of partial body training are both physical and mental as shown in the following validations.

Stopping Breath and Bodily Ki Flow through Mental Opposition

For example, if one takes a fighting pose and psyches oneself up by saying "I'm gonna do this!", then that person will be weak and their extended arm can be pushed down as per the illustration. The body actually knows it cannot resist the downward force, no matter how much one says "I'm gonna do this! - and fights against the arm being

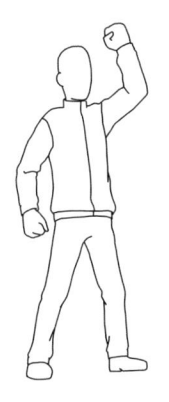
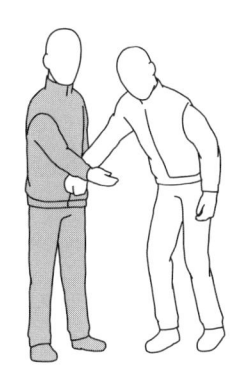

1. Taking a fighting pose and saying "I'm gonna do this!"   **2. The person is weak.**

taken down. This is because saying such words creates an oppositional disunity of heart and body and the body becomes weak.

The common pursuit of strength through muscle training is an underlying cause of this oppositional body structure. It may be difficult to understand this opposition through logic or the brain, but it will be clear through direct experience in the body. At Dou Juku, various validations are used to allow one to deepen an understanding through the body of the reality of this opposition. In addition, one learns that if the heart is harmonious, the mind and body can unify and overcome opposition. What is important is learning the mechanism for self-elevation, as opposed to competition, and striving to unlock the latent power human beings naturally possess. In this way, one can gain true self confidence.

The Normal Consciousness Hidden in Everyday Life that Stops Body Breathing

Everyday Consciousness that Stops Body Breathing:
1) Taiiku Suwari

There are many causes hidden in daily life for the stoppage of body breathing and ki flow. One example is taiiku suwari, which is a type of sitting style used by children in Japanese schools. One can understand why taiiku suwari stops the body breathing when a comparison is made with seiza, a traditional sitting style which means proper sitting. One can be easily knocked over when pushed from the side when sitting in taiiku suwari. But one is strong and not easily

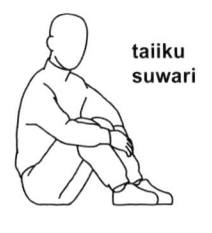

taiiku suwari

knocked down when sitting in seiza. In addition, one can easily validate that one is weak when standing up after sitting in taiiku suwari and strong after sitting in seiza.

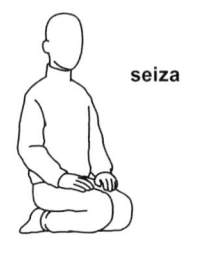

seiza

As mentioned before with the standing bow validations, the body is provisioned naturally from the outset with the capacity to respond optimally to various conditions via the unified structure of its 37 trillions cells and the 24000 strands of DNA in each cell. Sitting seiza properly provides the foundation for drawing out this power. Taiiku suwari, at its root core, destroys it.

According to the author, Toshiharu Takeuchi, taiiku suwari was introduced in Japanese schools for the first time in 1958. Japanese people from before that time had no experience with taiiku suwari as a sitting style. It has became a popular way of sitting in schools throughout Japan ever since because it purportedly helped children to concentrate and fidget less in class. But it was implemented without thought from the child's perspective.

Taiiku suwari has become a standard style of sitting in schools since its introduction, but it is most regrettable that its harmful effects have not even once been investigated. As made clear in the validations discussed, this posture of sitting immediately weakens the child by stopping the child's body breathing and ki flow. And rather than

promoting concentration, it actually inhibits the child's ability to focus.

It is said that children today get easily distracted and cannot concentrate. And to what cause can these weaknesses be attributed? Once again it would be good to investigate them in reference to the validations described above.

Everyday Consciousness that Stops Body Breathing:
2) Warm Up Exercises.

The warm up exercises done in schools and in public places all over Japan are well conceived as partial body exercises. But they are another matter from the perspective of whole body breathing. The difference will be made clear through experience using various validating examples.

Typical warm ups presented on Japanese radio stretch the body to the side. These exercises stretch the hip and side muscles and are believed to stimulate the digestive organs. But when one is pushed from the side while doing these exercises one can easily be knocked over. And this instability when pushed from the side comes from a lack of body breathing and ki flow in the body.

To change this side bend into an exercise where the body breath is flowing, place both hands above the head with the palms facing toward each other as in the illustration above. In contrast to the side bend before, the person is now strong and stable when pushed from the side.

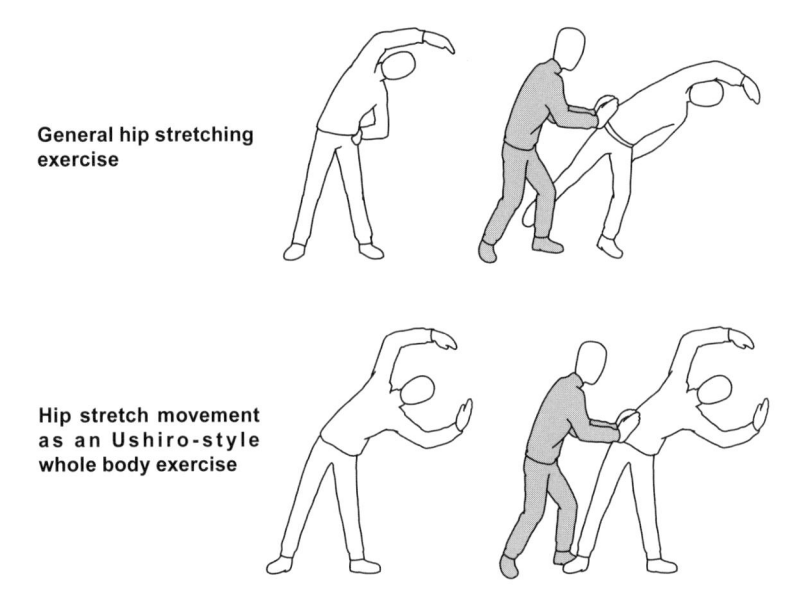

General hip stretching exercise

Hip stretch movement as an Ushiro-style whole body exercise

As in this example, the important thing is the flow of breath through the body. Doing exercises where ki is flowing makes the body stronger. Another radio warm up exercise is jumping in place. This exercise is supposed to be good for stimulating the thigh muscles, improving blood flow, and lowering stress. But whether it really has these effects and can be validated is another matter.

First, one puts one's legs together and jumps in place as per the radio warm up exercise. Then, to check the change in the body, someone firmly grabs the arm of the person jumping. The person who was jumping tries to throw in place but cannot throw the person grabbing. Next, the person tries jumping the Ushiro-style way, which is to start the jump a few times on the toes and then gradually return to a normal jump. When the person does the jumping in this manner, the

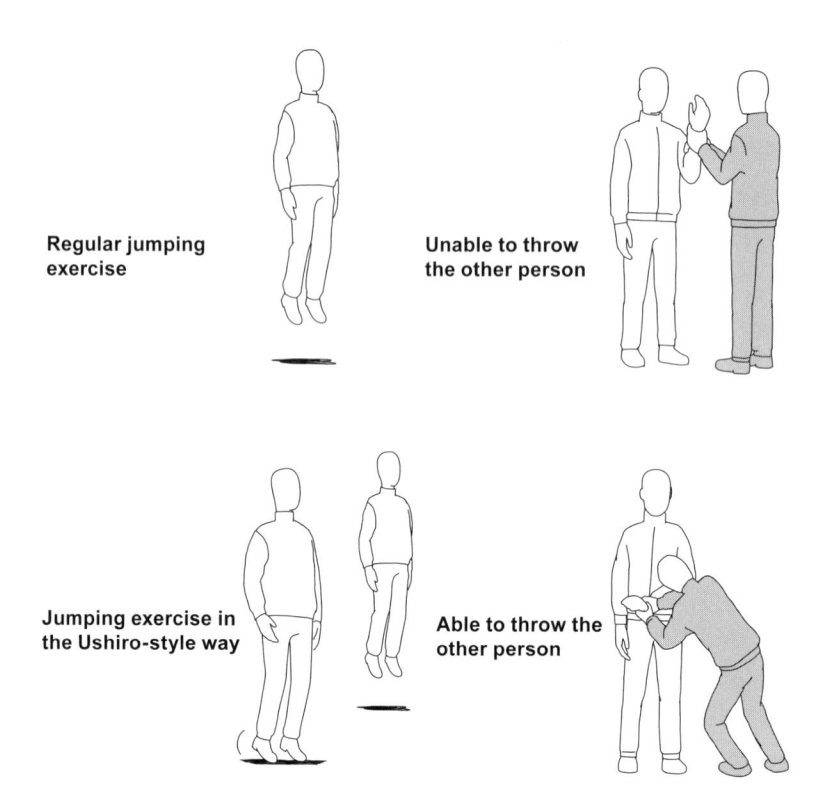

Regular jumping exercise

Unable to throw the other person

Jumping exercise in the Ushiro-style way

Able to throw the other person

throw can be executed with a surprising amount of power.

Why is there such a difference in result? It is because the body-part-based strengthening resulting from the radio warm ups and muscle training are not related to bringing out the power of living beings. Living beings must first have whole body ki flow for their power to manifest. Living beings cannot attain their power without first becoming whole body through the flow of ki.

Warm ups such as upper body side bends and jumping in place are partial body exercises that completely destroy the body. But if they

are done in the Ushiro-style manner, the body can return to its original condition and become strong again. For this reason, Ushiro-style exercises are also called recovery exercises.

Everyday Consciousness that Stops Body Breathing:
3) Not Breathing from the Heart

The flow or lack of breath in the body is heavily influenced by the manner of one's heart. The quality of body breath and heaviness will vary depending on whether your heart is generous and caring toward others or isolated and caring only toward oneself. For example, suppose one decided they could drive past and ignore a person in need on the

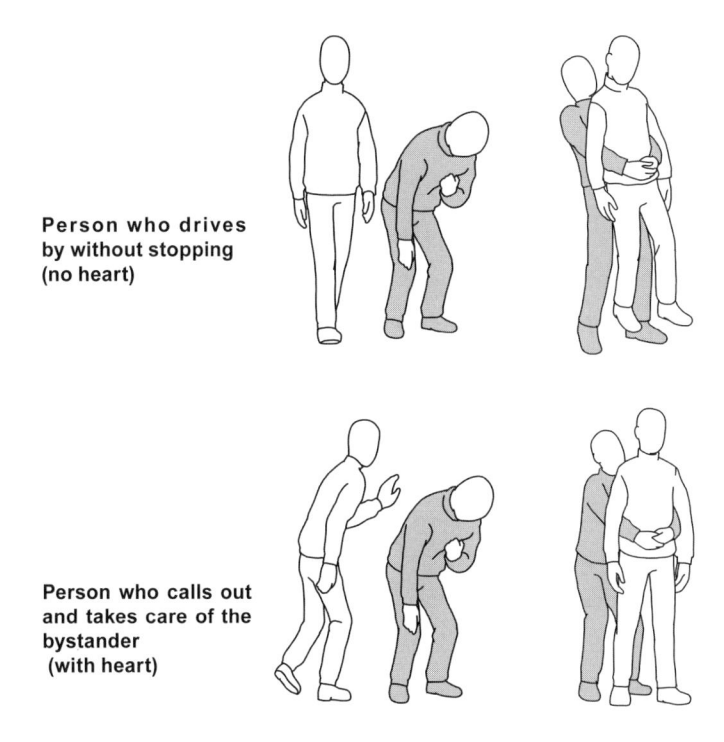

Person who drives by without stopping (no heart)

Person who calls out and takes care of the bystander (with heart)

side of the road. If the driver were then lifted from behind, he would be surprising light and easy to lift.

But if that same person were to instead walk up to the person in need asking what is wrong, that same person would be much heavier than before when lifted from behind.

Without heart, the body breathing stops and the body becomes light. With heart, the body breathing happens naturally and the body becomes heavy as ki is flowing.

This distinction will become clear when it is put into practice. The invisible condition of the heart affects the body as can be seen in these clear examples.

In this manner, the way of the heart makes for a heavy or light body, and even if it is invisible from the outside, the body always provides a response in accord with the heart.

That is, if breath and ki are running through the body allowing harmony with others and the outer environment, the body will attain its natural strength through the whole body condition where the body is heavy and stable.

Whole body is the condition in which the body can breathe, ki flows, and each part is connected together. And in this state, injury and fatigue are rare. In modern day sports, which focuses on increasing power and flexibility through western style warm ups, the body as a

whole does not become naturally strong. The real warm up is not one which acts on body parts, but one which must act on the cells of the entire body.

Ushiro-style whole body warm ups is a method that establishes the whole body condition allowing ki to flow.

Returning to the Body's Original Breathing

Ushiro-style breathing is not a partial body exercise program focusing on specific body part methods from the chest, stomach or tanden but rather a return to the whole body enabling us to take in the original power we possess as living beings. The important thing is experiencing whether or not ki is flowing in the body suffused with breath and orienting oneself toward a return to the original body within.

The body in its natural state does not get stuck or stiff and can move freely. Its separate parts come together as one and ki begins to flow. In this way, one can be aware of the difference in the body when ki is flowing or not. The understanding that "oh, this is how the natural body feels!" is the first step.

And this return to the natural body becomes the base for bringing out our latent energy within. It is a breathing method that makes for a body without openings and that transmits the hidden secrets of martial arts. It is our hope that through this book many people will have the opportunity to return to the natural breath of the body.

Reference video for the book
Please use the QR code or URL to access

Ushiro-style breathing and verification methods

Pass: usb005e

https://www.dou-shuppan.com/movie_ushiro-style-breathing/